JOSS GUIN

GATEWAYS TO HEALTH

KARMA YOGA

BRINGING YOGA INTO YOUR DAILY LIFE

WATKINS PUBLISHING

LONDON

This edition published in the UK 2009 by
Watkins Publishing, Sixth Floor, Castle House,
75–76 Wells Street, London W1T 3QH

Conceived, created and designed by Duncan Baird Publishers

1 3 5 7 9 10 8 6 4 2

Designed by Clare Thorpe
Commissioned artwork by Conny Jude (www.connyjude.com)
and Art-4

Printed and bound in Great Britain

British Library Cataloguing-in-Publication Data Available

ISBN: 978-1-906787-18-9

www.watkinspublishing.co.uk

Contents

Introduction

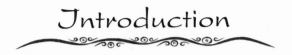

Karma and Yoga

Yoga is the mother of all the Eastern methods of self-development. Its origins are lost in prehistory, but we know that in India, 5,000-year-old statues have been found showing figures in yoga poses. Buddha practised yoga, and the yoga word for meditation, *dhyana*, is the root of the Japanese word *Zen*.

The word yoga has become synonymous with the poses that give so many health benefits, but yoga actually means union. Yoga is any exercise that promotes union between your body, mind, spirit, and the world around you.

This book teaches simple yoga poses, breathing techniques and meditations that anyone can do. It also provides a gateway between yoga as an exercise and Karma Yoga which you can practise all the time.

Karma means action, so Karma Yoga is the

'Yoga of Action'. It is a method designed for those who do not have the time or the temperament for devotion, for austerities or for philosophical study.

It was first taught about 2,500 years ago to a king who was sick of his duties in life. The king's guru said that renouncing your duties and becoming a monk is one way to find peace, but that it is better to do your duty and make what you do Yoga.

Another way of thinking of Karma is as your emotional baggage and habits; it is your actions, but it is also the result of past actions. Emotional baggage and habits stay with us because we unconsciously keep doing the same things out of the same motives. In a way we are trapped and it is this trap that causes all our stress and suffering. The only way out is to start acting consciously, and that is what Karma Yoga helps you to do.

The Benefits of Karma Yoga

Learning Karma Yoga through the medium of yoga poses is ideal because you get the benefits of the exercise, as well as the benefits of Karma Yoga in your daily life.

Yoga poses always give increased strength and flexibility. They can balance hormones, and best of all yoga helps to relieve and even prevent stress. Most people, however, find that the benefits of a yoga workout fade in a day or two.

So in this book we start with the pose or meditation, and then go on to use it as a symbol for a virtue to develop in daily life. These are not virtues for virtue's sake, but are practical ways of improving your life and obtaining peace. For example, by developing courage and truthfulness in The Warrior pose (pages 18–23) you can prevent being taken advantage of in life.

This focus on a virtue is also designed to make you more aware in your daily life. For example, if you are focusing on peace and you get angry, then you will be more aware. When you have that awareness you can check your motives and methods and escape your habits.

Practising Karma Yoga in your daily life can

also give you a lot of energy; many people find they get a lot more done. Normally we either work on autopilot or are thinking about what we will get out of what we are doing; this stagnates or disperses our energy. But, if the virtue you are working on makes you focused and aware of only what you are doing, then your energy is likewise focused.

Finally, through Karma Yoga you can achieve unity. This happens as you become aware that the best motives go beyond you. As you slowly revise your motives they stop being about you, you are united with everything. In that state you experience the greatest happiness possible.

Ashram and Guru

Traditionally, Karma Yoga was practised in an *ashram* and under the guidance of a *guru*. Ashram means a place of hard spiritual work, like a monastery, and is usually controlled by a guru or teacher. Guru literally means 'the one who enlightens'. The teacher would set chores and their disciples would try to do those chores without ego and in full awareness. The disciples would surrender their ego to the guru.

These ideas can be very useful in your practice of Karma Yoga. You may not have a guru or time to spend in an ashram but you can choose to view the world in a positive and helpful manner. You can treat the whole world as your ashram, a place where you have gone to uncover your nature. You can also view your life as a guru, a sometimes harsh but always loving teacher. This attitude can greatly help your practice of Yoga and your life in general.

How to Practise Karma Yoga

Yoga is a little different from other kinds of exercise. Attitude is as important as technique. Practise with an empty stomach, use the toilet and wash first so that you feel fresh and light. Try to practise at the same time each day, and whenever you practise, spend a few moments consciously setting aside your worries and plans to tune in to how your body feels. Treat each exercise as a journey you start anew each time you practise. Find your initial limits and never strain, and over time expand and explore those limits, growing in strength, flexibility and understanding.

Once you are comfortable with the movement of the pose or meditation, start to contemplate it as a symbol for its corresponding virtue while you practise. This series of yoga exercises has been chosen because they best symbolize the ten virtues that are the foundation of yoga practice. These are Peace, Truth, Honesty, Control, Freedom, Cleanliness, Contentment, Willpower, Insight and Surrender. For example, The Cleansing Breath (page 44) is great for soothing your nervous system, but in addition it is used here as a symbol for Cleanliness.

Once you are comfortable with the pattern of breathing in The Cleansing Breath, you can then consider, while practising, the corresponding virtue of Cleanliness and what needs cleaning out in your life.

Following each exercise in this book is a further practice under the heading 'In Daily Life'. These are what help you to take the power of yoga beyond the mat. They provide a focus to help make you more conscious in everything you experience. Avoid trying more than one of these at a time, and take a relaxed but determined attitude to each.

The ten exercises can be practised independently or as a series, so you can tailor your approach to your own needs. For the best results I suggest doing the first five in the morning and the second five after your working day is done, but focus on mastering just one virtue each week.

You can take the initiative in your yoga practice, experiment and keep a record to refer back to, study books by great yoga teachers to broaden your knowledge, and best of all, go and study with great yoga teachers.

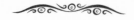

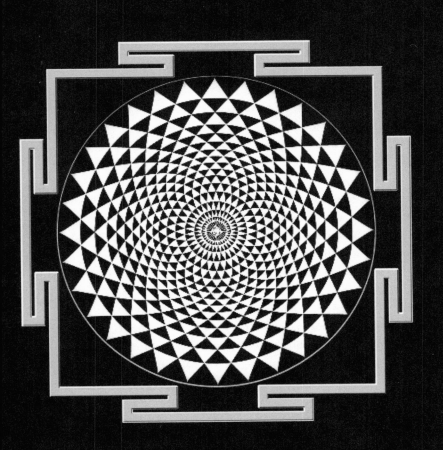

The Exercises

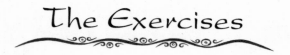

The Hare and the Cobra

This combination of poses will improve the mobility of your spine and will also aid the functioning of your adrenal glands, which produce adrenalin to aid your fight-or-flight response when you are under threat. The Hare is alert and ready to run, while the Cobra hisses and strikes out. For that reason this exercise is a good symbol for developing peace or non-violence, the first virtue.

1 Start in a kneeling position with your palms on your knees, back straight, and eyes closed. If you have trouble kneeling, place a cushion between your calves and thighs. Be calm but alert like a Hare that has caught wind of danger.

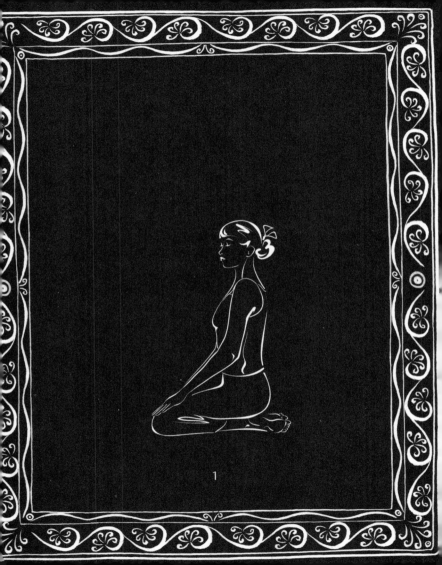

1

2   Inhale as you lift your arms above your head. Time the movement so that you start to inhale as you begin to move, and finish the movement as your inhalation is complete. Avoid straining or artificial pauses in your movements or breathing.

3   Exhale as you bend forwards at the waist while keeping your lower body still. Gently tense your abdomen and perineum as you move to strengthen and support your core. Place your palms on the ground as far forward as you can without lifting from your seat. Allow the movement to help empty your lungs. Remain in this position for a few peaceful breaths. Feel how your abdomen is massaged by your breath because of the posture.

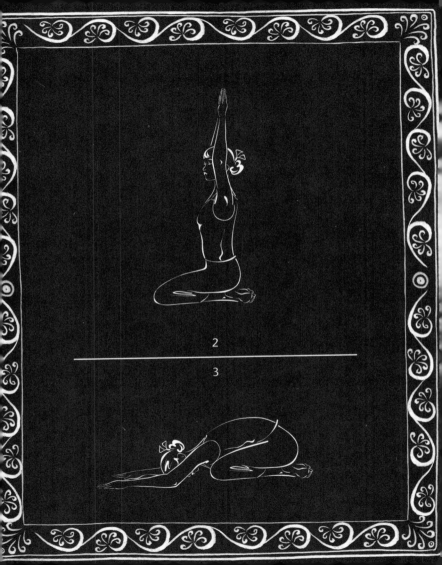

2

3

4   Inhale as you move your weight onto your hands.
     Pull up your pelvic floor as you glide forwards
     first then arch up like a striking cobra. You may
     need to move your hands forward a little first, but
     keep your lower legs still.

     Reverse back through the poses to the beginning,
     and repeat three to five times.

In Daily Life

Focus on developing Peace in your life by noting
what makes you angry or causes you to harm
others or yourself. When you feel anger, you
can use the energy it gives you constructively, for
example to complete some mundane task.

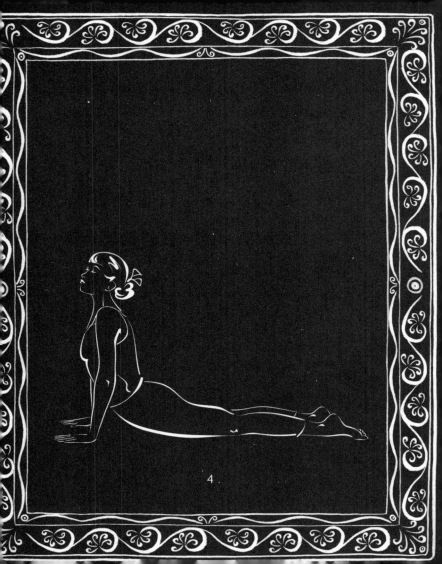

4

The Warrior

This pose is inspired by a mighty hero. As you practise, feel and know you have the courage to stand up for yourself and those you love. Courage gives you the freedom to be true to yourself. So this pose is used as a symbol for truthfulness.

I Start by standing tall and straight with your feet together and your arms by your sides. Your big toes should be touching, but your heels should be slightly apart. Expand your chest a little and tuck your chin in slightly. Feel a sense of lift starting from the ground and going up through your body, as you become conscious of your whole body from toe to head. Avoid locking your knees. Then feel a sense of relaxation descending from your head down to the ground so that you are not standing stiffly.

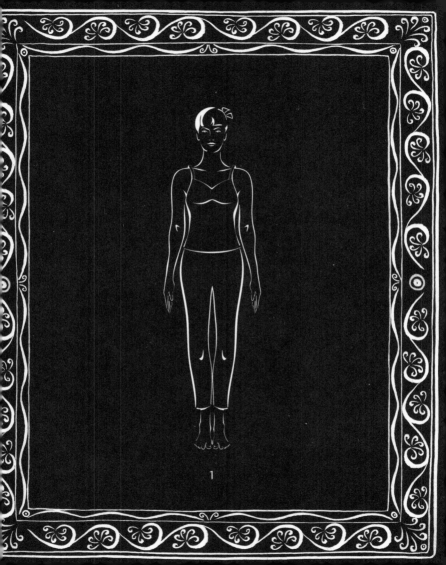

2 Now inhale as you step your feet out smoothly and raise your arms to shoulder height, palms down. Keep your shoulders down. If possible, finish with your feet beneath your palms with your toes still pointing forwards.

3 Breathing normally, transfer a little of your weight onto your right leg. Turning on your left heel, turn your left foot out so that your toes are pointing to your left. Move slowly and smoothly to avoid losing balance. Allow your torso to follow the movement slightly but avoid moving your right hip. Turn your head to gaze at the fingertips of your left hand.

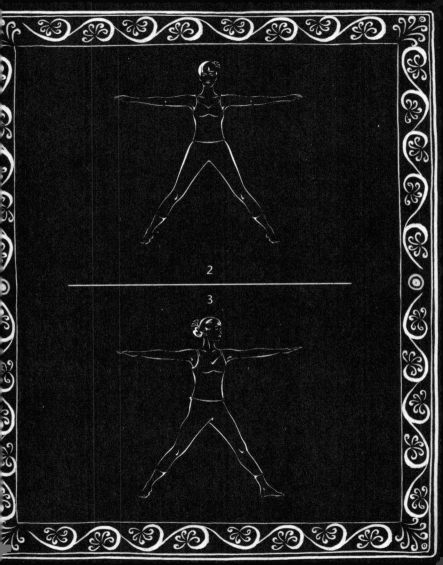

2

3

4 In the final pose bend your left leg until the thigh is almost parallel to the floor and your left knee is over your ankle pointing towards your toes. Use your strength to hold the pose and breathe naturally for up to a minute.

Repeat on the right side, then shake out your limbs and do the pose on each side once more.

In Daily Life

To work towards being truthful to yourself in daily life, try tallying up any time you accidentally or habitually tell a lie or hide your true feelings. Try and reduce your score daily. This helps you become more conscious of what you say, and it can help you to remember that your unconscious mind records everything you say, believes it all to be true, and acts on it.

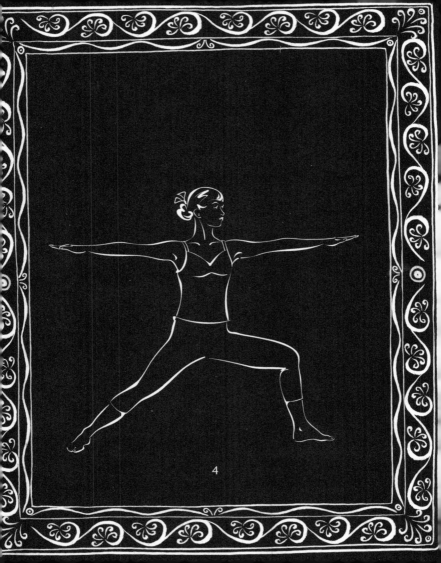

4

Rising Up

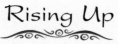

These poses are great to warm you up and strengthen your legs and core. As you rise up from the forward bend to standing feel a sense of upliftment, as if rising above your animal nature.

This exercise is about honesty. One major cause of stress is taking more than you are due, being a borrower or being a lender. Not just financially but emotionally too.

1   Begin standing with your feet together.

2   Inhale as you raise your arms above your head.

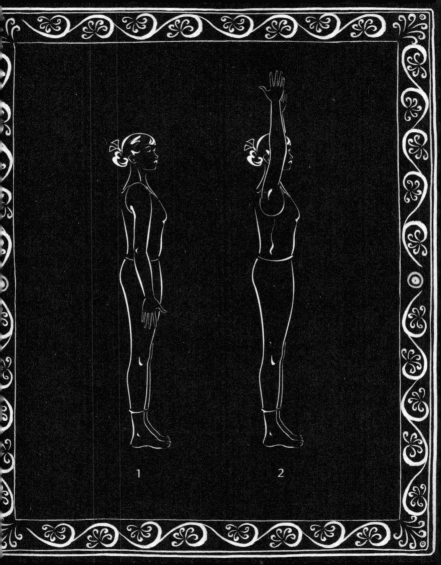

3 Then bend your knees and lower your torso as if sitting into a chair. You can tuck your tailbone under slightly to engage your abdominal muscles.

4 Now exhale as you bend forwards at the waist and place your hands on the floor or hold your ankles. Straighten your legs as much as you can. Look back towards your legs.

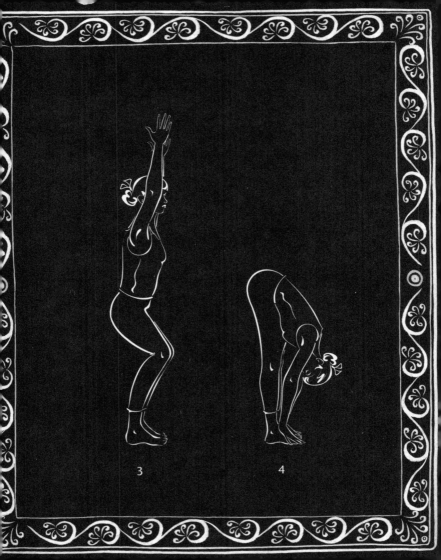

3   4

5 From that position, bend your knees a little and use strength in your gut and legs to stand up straight as you inhale back to position 2, and then exhale to position 1. Be like a monkey or half man learning to be fully human, and to stand upright and honest. Practise three to five rounds.

In Daily Life

To carry honesty into your daily life, spend a few days answering the following questions to yourself. What have I ever taken that I have not earned? When have I made someone else indebted? How could I put things right?

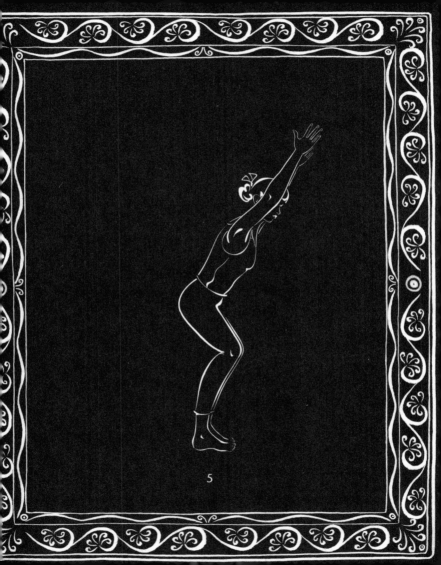

5

The Boat

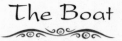

This pose is great for abdominal strength, and teaches the secret of *tense and release*. It relieves tension patterns and gives you energy back.

The Boat is used here as a symbol for control, especially of your vital energy. When you have lots of lusts you waste vital energy chasing them. Just like with tension patterns in your body the best way to deal with them is to be aware and let them go.

1 Start this pose lying on your back with your arms by your sides and legs together. Have a pillow under your head. Your eyes can be open or closed throughout this exercise.

2 Inhale as you lift your straight legs and upper body an inch or two off the ground.

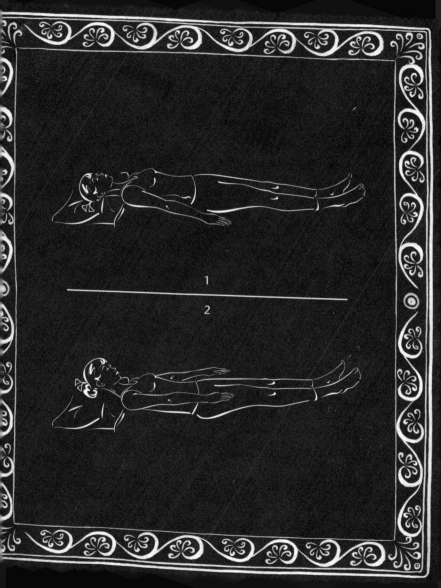

1

2

3   Holding your breath, tense all your muscles. Tense your face, hands, feet and abdomen, concentrating especially on pulling up your pelvic floor. Try and find the normally tense areas of your body and tense them a little more.

4   When you need to exhale, do so all at once with a sound like 'Ah' and let your body fall back to the floor as you release all that tension. Repeat three to five times.

In Daily Life

To control a lust/desire and regain all the vital energy it consumes, first exaggerate it in your mind until it seems the most important thing, and then trivialize it until you can barely remember why it moved you. Keep expanding and contracting the desire until you realize the desire is all in your mind.

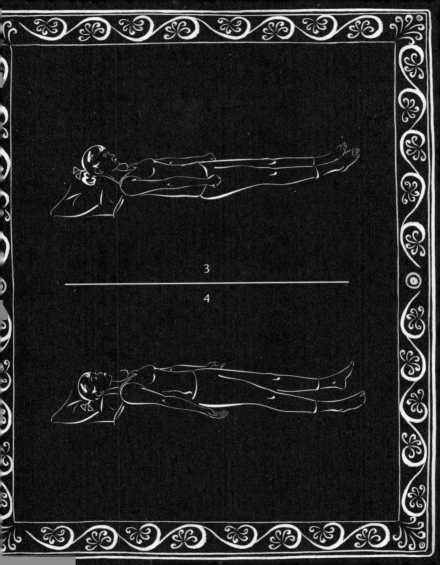

3

4

Freeing Movements

These simple movements relieve subtle tensions around the joints, giving you freer movement. We use these exercises as a symbol for freedom, especially from attachment to possessions.

Move consciously and slowly and in time with your breath. Do each movement three–five times, or if rotating a joint practise three–five times in each direction.

1   Start sitting with your legs out in front of you, back straight and palms resting on your thighs. You can sit on a cushion to avoid your lower back slumping. Inhale and spread your toes out.

2   Exhale and make fists with your feet.

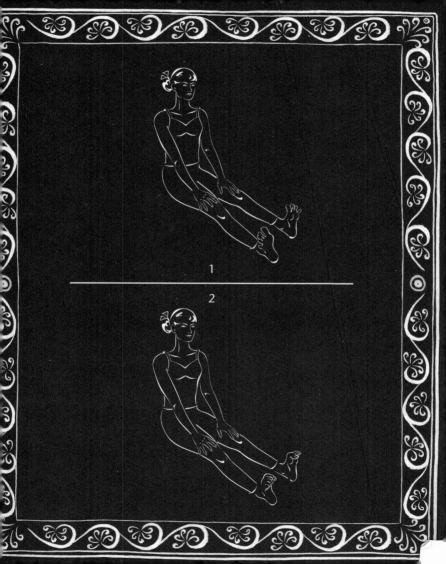

1

2

3 Move your feet slightly apart to rotate your ankles without moving the rest of your legs. Make the biggest circles you can. Move in time with your breath, inhaling as your foot comes towards you. Isolate the movement in your ankles and feel the effect all the way up to your hips.

4 Hold under one thigh with clasped hands and point your toes. Exhale as you lift your knee up towards your chest and simultaneously move your toes towards your shin. Then inhale as you straighten your leg and point your toes. Practise with both right and left legs.

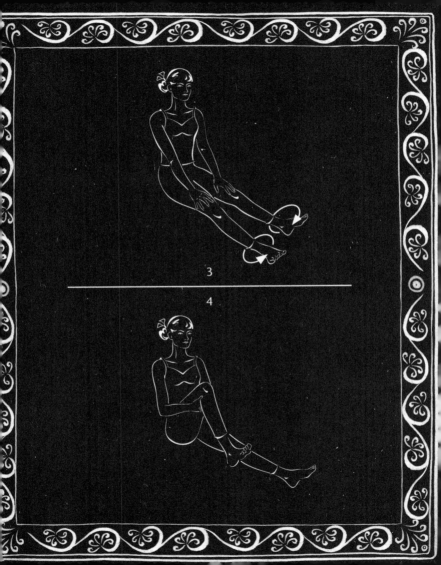

3

4

5 Lift your arms up to shoulder height and extend them out in front of you. Inhale as you spread out your fingers, and exhale as you make fists with the thumbs inside your fingers.

6 Rotate your wrists equal times in each direction, inhaling as the fists go up.

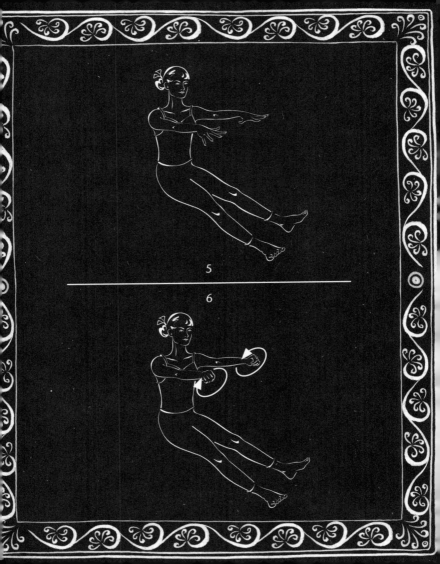

5

6

7   Stretching your arms in front of you with your palms up, inhale. Exhale as you bend your elbows, touching your fingers to your shoulders, and inhale as your straighten your arms, palms facing up.

8   Touching your shoulders with your fingertips and moving your elbows out to the side, rotate your shoulders by making big circles with your elbows. Inhale as you lift your elbows up and over and exhale as you bring your elbows down and together at the front. Do three circles and then reverse direction for another three rotations.

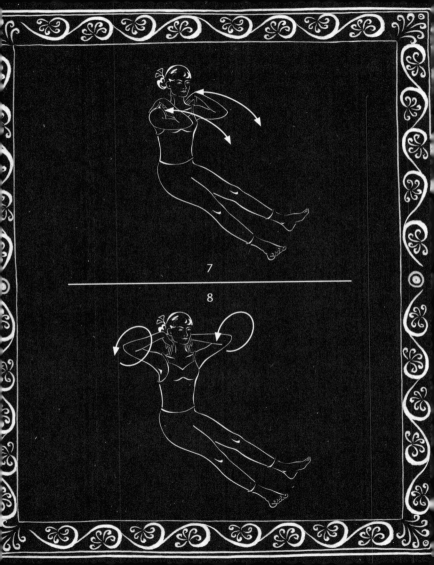

7

8

9   Slowly stand up with your feet facing forwards, shoulder width apart, put your hands on your hips and move your waist in circles starting small and getting bigger. Do three circles in each direction.

10 Still standing with your pelvis facing forwards, relax your arms and turn your torso and head to the left. Let your right arm swing across your chest, while your left arm swings behind your back. Reverse these positions as you swing back to the right.

In Daily Life

To focus on freedom from attachments, contemplate all the relationships you have with the people, places and possessions in your life. Imagine the connection as a line of force. Instead of being tied by these lines, imagine returning the force of these lines into your body and tying them off at each end.

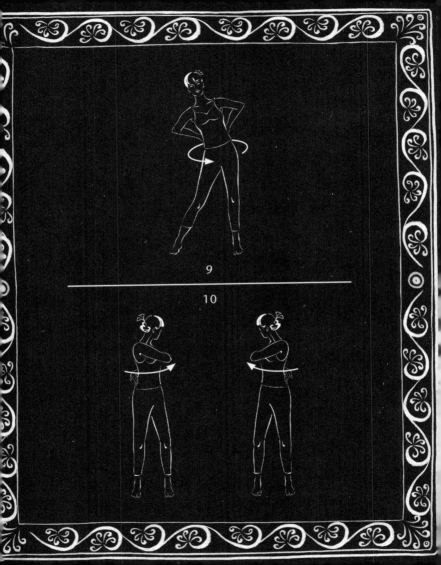

9

10

The Cleansing Breath

This is a powerful cleansing exercise for your entire nervous system. Keeping your body, mind, energy, and environment clean is an important practice and an easy one to focus on in your daily life.

Sit comfortably on the floor or on a chair with your back straight, and close your eyes. Feel how your body expands as you inhale, and contracts as you exhale. Expand from the abdomen up, and contract from the chest down. Let your breath be the same length in and out. Lift your right hand and rest your middle and index fingers on your brow. Rest your thumb on your right nostril, and your ring finger on your left nostril so you can control which nostril air passes through.

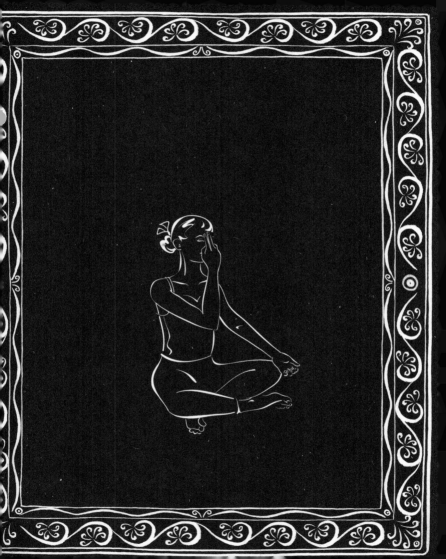

After you exhale, close your right nostril. Inhale through your left nostril imagining cool fresh moonlight filling your body. Close your left nostril and open your right nostril, exhaling stale sunlight. Without changing nostrils inhale fresh warm sunlight through your right nostril. Close your right nostril, open your left nostril, and exhale cold clammy moonlight. Repeat the round up to five times without straining.

In Daily Life

Imagination and symbols help to tell your subconscious mind what you want to achieve. So when focusing on cleanliness in your daily life, imagine your shower cleansing your whole system, your food being filled with pure energy, your in-breath being pure, and your out-breath carrying away toxins and tension. When you do housework, imagine white light shining where you have cleaned.

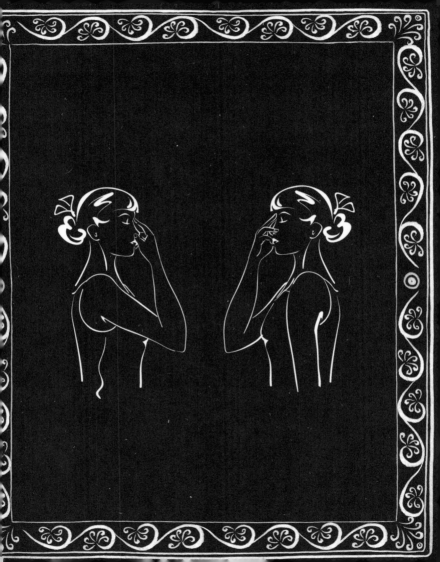

The Gesture of Peace

This *mudra*, or gesture, can create a strong sense of peace in your body. Regular practice helps prevent stress. We use it here as a symbol of contentment.

1 Close your eyes throughout this exercise. Sit cross-legged with your back straight and your hands resting in your lap, palms up and fingers touching. Relax as you exhale.

2 As you inhale, lift your hands up along the centre of your body, imagining a tide of gentle white light filling your body wherever your hands pass.

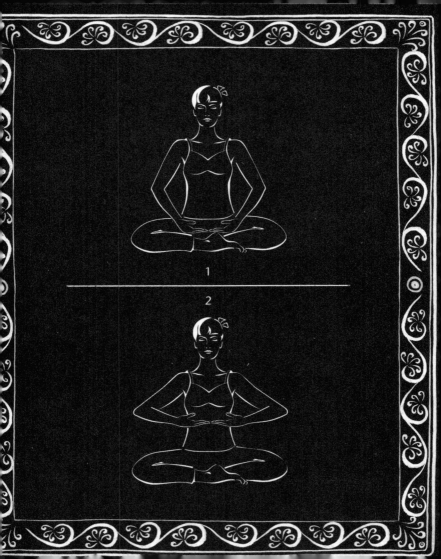

1

2

3   As your hands reach your throat spread them out
    to the sides, imagining the tide of light continuing
    up into your head. Pause a moment, emanating
    peace to the whole world.

4   As you exhale, lower your arms, withdrawing the
    tide of light back to your feet. Repeat the exercise
    five times, moving more slowly each time and
    making the light more intense.

In Daily Life

To focus on contentment in daily life, practise
curbing the habit of unnecessary worrying. Try
to catch yourself when you are wishing the past
was different, or the world was different, or you
were different. When you do, review all that is
wonderful and good about the present moment,
and try to resolve any problems that your worry
made you aware of in a positive manner.

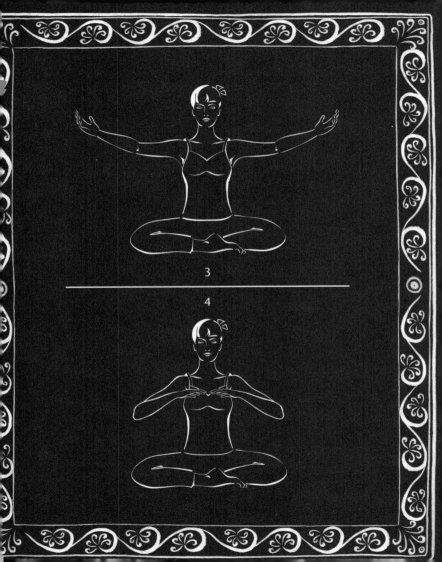

3

4

Concentration

Mental energy can be concentrated just like light. When light is concentrated it becomes a laser that can cut through anything, just as your concentrated willpower can move any obstacle.

Sit comfortably on a chair or the floor and close your eyes, letting your body settle until you are as still as a statue. Open your eyes and gaze intently at the centre of the image opposite. Whenever something distracts you, even if your focus changes, return your gaze. If you need to rest your eyes for a moment, keep a mental image of the *yantra* in your head. Practise for two minutes and increase a little each day up to ten minutes.

In Daily Life

As you start each task throughout your day, mentally declare it as your one focus. If your mind strays away from what you are doing, congratulate yourself each time you re-focus.

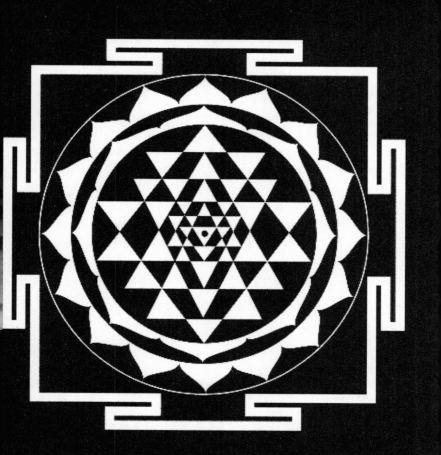

Inner Quiet

This is the name of a meditation that gives you great insight into your own nature and the way you interact with the world. Knowing yourself is one of the most important things in life. Not knowing yourself is the fundamental cause of confusion and anxiety. So this exercise is a symbol and practice for insight.

Start by practising this meditation for five to ten minutes in the pose, and then slowly extending the time as you get into it. Then carry the ability to witness yourself out into daily life, practising the meditation while you work and play.

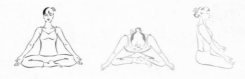

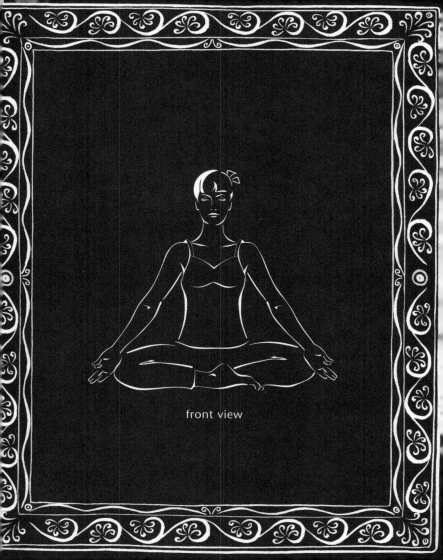

front view

The Posture

The Auspicious Pose is the easiest yoga meditation position for beginners. The idea is to be like a pyramid; note the triangular shape from any angle. Respect the natural curves of your spine, ensure your chin is tucked in to open the back of your neck, and your head is central, but avoid inclining your head.

You can use a cushion to elevate your position so that your bottom is higher than your knees. Fold your legs in so one heel presses your perineum and the other presses the first ankle. Sit towards the front of your sitting bones and feel a gentle sense of lift through your body. Rest the back of your wrists on your knees with your arms straight and your shoulders relaxed; you can also touch the tips of your index fingers in to the base of your thumbs.

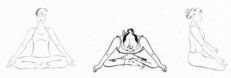

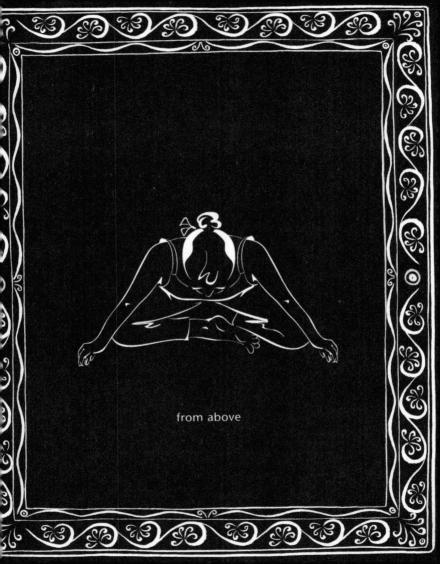

from above

The Meditation

Sitting in The Auspicious Pose, become aware of any sounds you can hear. Be aware if your mind labels the sounds, or if you judge them. Witness your mind's reactions to the sounds you hear. Then be aware of the inner quiet that lies behind your perception of noise.

After a little while leave the sounds and just be aware of any thoughts that come into your mind and again notice if you are judging your thoughts. You are practising your ability to witness your own experience, and the quiet that lies behind it.

In Daily Life

To gain insight, practise this meditation whenever you can, and wherever you are: queuing for the bus; walking home; or going to sleep. Ask yourself, 'Am I my thoughts and experiences? Who am I?'

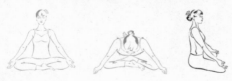

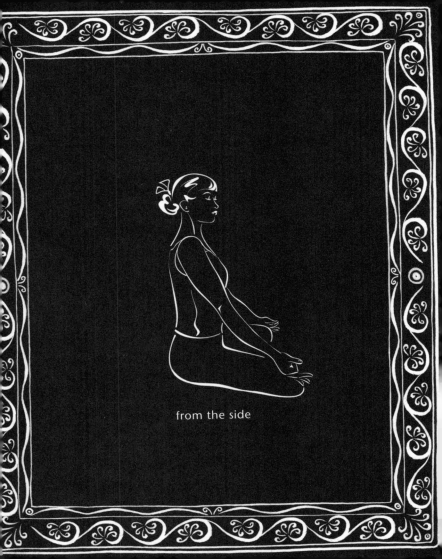

from the side

Deep Relaxation

To relax requires the ability to be conscious and to let go. As you learn to surrender physical tension, you can learn to surrender mental tension too. So this exercise is a symbol for surrender, especially of the ego. Ego is what separates you from living in harmony with the world.

Start by lying on you back with a pillow under your head and knees, arms away from your body, palms up and legs apart, letting the feet fall out to the sides. Place a blanket over your body and close your eyes. Once you are comfortable, keep still for the whole exercise.

Now move your attention slowly around your body, mentally touching the following points. Start at your brow, go down to your throat, down the right arm, touching shoulder, elbow and wrist and hand, back up your right arm and back to your throat. Next go down your left arm, touching the same points.

Continue back up the left arm and from your throat down the centre of your body, touching the centre of your chest, your navel and your pelvis. Then go down the right leg, touching the hip, knee, ankle and foot, back up the right leg, across the pelvis and down the left leg, touching the same points. Finally, go up the body, touching your pelvis, navel, chest, throat, and back to your brow.

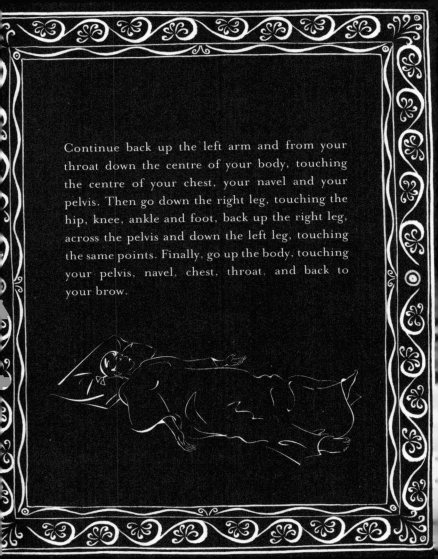

Mentally touch each point for the length of a breath, and as you exhale let go of any tensions gathered there. If you fall asleep, when you wake resume the exercise from where you left off. Finally, before you finish expand your attention to encompass your whole body and take a little time to come round gently before getting up.

In Daily Life

To practise surrender, choose occasions when you are working hard and expending effort, especially if it is not going as you expected or intended. Surrender the work and whatever comes of it to something beyond yourself. Do this with a loving attitude, like you would if the work was for someone you love.